ALKALINE DIET

The Complete Guide for Alkaline Diet and Achieve Health Benefits and Lose Weight in a Healthy Natural Way

Nancy Franklin

Published by David Kruse Publishing House

Alkaline Diet: The Complete Guide for Alkaline Diet and Achieve Health Benefits and Lose Weight in a Healthy Natural Way

ISBN 978-1-989744-00-0

Legal & Disclaimer

held liable for any errors or omissions. Changes are periodically made to this book. You must consult your doctor or get professional medical advice before using any of the suggested remedies, techniques, or information in this book.

Upon using the information contained in this book, you agree to hold harmless the Author from and against any damages, costs, and expenses, including any legal fees potentially resulting from the application of any of the information provided by this guide. This disclaimer applies to any damages or injury caused by the use and application, whether directly or indirectly, of any advice or information presented, whether for breach of contract, tort, negligence, personal injury, criminal intent, or under any other cause of action.

You agree to accept all risks of using the information presented inside this book. You need to consult a professional medical practitioner in order to ensure you are both able and healthy enough to participate in this program.

TABLE OF CONTENTS

Part - 1

Introduction

First off all, thank you for deciding to grab a copy of this book. It is my hope that you will enjoy reading and implementing it!

Recipes of the alkaline diet inside this book are quick and easy to make and they will give you huge amounts of energy throughout your day. They are suitable for all events, and they provide a range of different tastes, and they are also full of nutritious goods such a vitamins and minerals which serve to recover the cells inside your body. This enables you to have more life energy, lower inflammations, as well as help you with rapid weight loss.

Inside this book, you will find easy, practicable, actionable steps which also make it fun for yourself. There are a wide range of recipes great for everyone, not just for health enthusiasts or vegans and vegetarians, but anyone can find tremendous benefit from it.

Once again, I want to thank you for grabbing a copy of this book. Now lets begin on your alkaline diet journey!

Delicious Butternut Squash Soup

Servings: **6**
Ingredients:
Pepper
Himalayan salt
Optional: a few drops of Stevia to sweeten
½ tsp /2 ½ ml Cinnamon
2 14 oz. cans/784 g low-sodium vegetable broth
1 large chopped apple
¼ tsp /1 ¼ ml nutmeg
1 medium chopped butternut squash
3 medium chopped carrots
1 medium chopped onion
Chickpeas:

1/8 tsp /7/8 ml salt

¼ tsp /1 ¼ ml cinnamon

15 oz. can /420 g chickpeas

1 tbsp. /15 ml coconut oil

Instructions:

Add the fruits and vegetables to the slow cooker.

Top with the broth.

Set for six hours on low.

After the veggies are soft, puree everything with an immersion blender.

Stir in all the seasonings and add pepper and salt to your taste.

As the soup cooks, is the perfect time to fix the chickpeas.

The oven should be at 375.

Rinse the chickpeas and dry them.

Make sure to take off their skin.

Mix all the chickpea seasonings together and toss in the chickpeas.

Place them on a baking sheet and bake 40 to 45 minutes. Be sure to stir every 15 minutes.

Serve the soup with the chickpeas.

Tasty Spelt Porridge

Ingredients:

1 cup of filtered water

1/3 cup of flaked spelt

Powdered stevia or agave for sweetening

Cinnamon to taste

2-3 tablespoons of cranberries or cherries (dried)

¼ teaspoon of vanilla

Toppings: hemp nuts, raw nuts, blueberries, hazelnut and hemp milk.

Procedure:

Combine your first 6 ingredients and allow it to simmer for at least 3 to 4 minutes before transferring it to a shallow bowl.

Once done, sprinkle your toppings all over it.

Add your non-dairy milk (almond or hazelnut would work too).

Serve warm.

Yummy Alkaline Diet Avocado Peach Porridge

INGREDIENTS:

1 ripe peach

4 oz. gluten free porridge oats

3 tbsp. desiccated coconut

2 tbsp. chia seeds

2 cups of water

1/2 an avocado, finely sliced

Flaked almonds

INSTRUCTIONS:

•Cut the peach, remove the seed and slit into small square pieces.

•Place the peach cubes on a pan.

•Add the oats, desiccated coconut, chia seeds and half of the water to the pan

•Heat and bring to simmer on a medium flame.

•When the mixture thickens, add the remaining water and cook the porridge till ready.

•Peel the avocado, remove the seed and slice into half moon shapes.

• Serve into bowls and top with the avocado slices and flaked almonds.

Scrumptious Quinoa White Chili

Servings: **6 - 8**

Ingredients:

Lime wedges

Cilantro

2 15-oz. /420 g cans cannellini beans, drained

4 cups /960 ml low-sodium vegetable broth

1 tsp /5 ml salt

2 tsp /10 ml ground cumin

2 cloves garlic, minced

¼ tsp /1 ¼ ml paprika

¼ tsp /1 ¼ ml ground cloves

¾ cup /720 ml uncooked quinoa, rinsed with cold water, drained well

1 medium chopped onion

1 tsp /5 ml oregano

1 tbsp. /15 ml olive oil

2 medium poblano peppers

1 medium bell pepper, chopped

Tabasco sauce to taste

Instructions:

Roast the poblano first. Oven needs to be on broil.

Move oven rack as close to broiler as possible.

Wash and dry the pepper and put on baking sheet.

Put in oven on broil for two to three minutes until black.

Flip them over.

Cook until blackened and blistered.

Keep an eye on them: you want them blackened, not burnt.

Remove and place in brown paper bag to sweat.

Heat up a pan with oil.

Cook bell peppers and onions until soft. Add spices.

Deglaze pan with broth.

Pour into slow cooker.

Add rest of broth, quinoa, beans, and Tabasco.

Peel skin off poblano and remove stem. Chop and put into slow cooker. Mix together.

Allow to cook for about nine hours on low.

Taste and adjust seasonings.

Mouth Watering Power Smoothie
Ingredients:
1 ¼ of coconut water
½ cup of unsweetened almond milk
A cup of frozen blueberries
2/3 cup of frozen raspberries
2 tablespoons of agave or stevia
1 avocado, sliced
3 tablespoons of fresh coconut meat
½ a teaspoon of super greens powder
4 tablespoons of raw hemp nuts
2 tablespoons of omega 3 oil
Procedure:

Combine all of your ingredients in a blender.

Mince your raspberries and add some more coconut water if you think the consistency needs it.

Blend well until it becomes thick and creamy.

Yields 4 cups.

Heavenly Alkaline Diet Energy Enhancing Porridge

INGREDIENTS:

2 oz. oats

2 cups of water

1 ¾ cups water

1 tbsp. Bioglan Energy Boosting powder

1 tbsp. almond butter

1 tbsp. coconut oil

1 tsp. cinnamon

Coconut blossom or rice syrup to taste

Frozen berries to garnish

INSTRUCTIONS:

•Place the oats and 1 cup water in a pan on medium flame.

•Cook until the porridge is ready.

•Add the remaining water and the stir in the Bioglan energy boosting powder.

•Add the coconut oil, almond butter, cinnamon and stir until you obtain the desired consistency.

•Serve into bowls, add some syrup and garnish with the berries.

Irresistible Italian Bean Soup

Servings: 6

Ingredients:

Pepper

Salt

1 tbsp. /15 ml fennel seeds

2 tsp /10 ml oregano

¼ tsp /1 ¼ ml red pepper flakes

1 small chopped onion

2 celery ribs, chopped

3 medium chopped carrots

1 lb. /454 g dry Great Northern Beans

2 tsp /10 ml garlic powder

Instructions:

Add carrots, onions, celery, beans, spices except salt and pepper, and five cups cold water to cooker.

Set for five hours on high.

Add more water to give the soup the thickness you want. Add pepper and salt to taste. Serve and enjoy.

Delicious Spelt and Vanilla Vegan Pancakes

Ingredients:

1 cup of light spelt flour

1/8 teaspoon of fine Himalayan salt

2 tablespoon of aluminum free baking powder

1 cup of almond milk

1 tablespoon of maple syrup or stevia

1 ½ teaspoon of alcohol free vanilla

2 tablespoons of cold pressed sunflower oil

Coconut oil for greasing

Procedure:

Measure all of your dry ingredients in one bowl and the wet ones into a separate one.

Give each a stir before combining. Make sure it's mixed well and evenly.

Set this aside for at least 5 minutes and allow it to rise.

While waiting, prepare your open pan and brush on ¼ teaspoon of coconut oil on it, keeping the heat low.

Spoon your batter into this, forming 3 small pancakes. Cook for 3 minutes or until each side become golden.

Tasty Alkaline Diet Lemon Turmeric Pancakes

INGREDIENTS:

3.5 oz. gluten free flour

1 egg

1 cup rice milk

1 tsp. syrup – rice syrup, agave or coconut palm syrup

1 tsp. sunflower oil

1 inch fresh grated turmeric

1 lemon zest

INSTRUCTIONS:

•Whisk the egg with rice milk and sunflower oil in a bowl.

•Grate the turmeric and lemon into the bowl and mix it.

•Sieve the flower and add to the mixture slowly until you obtain the desired consistency.

•Heat a non-stick pan and apply oil onto the pan.

•Ladle some quantity of the mixture into the pan and spread evenly and thickly.

•Cook until the pan side of the pancake is golden brown and you can move the pancake with a spatula.

•Flip it over with the spatula and leave it until done.

•Make pancakes with the remaining batter, in the same manner.

•Serve with a drizzle of syrup and lemon juice.

Yummy Black Bean Stew

Servings: **6 - 8**
Ingredients:
Pepper
Salt
1 - 2 dried chipotle peppers
¾ cup /720 ml uncooked quinoa, rinsed
1 cinnamon stick
3 minced garlic cloves
1 chopped green bell pepper
7 cups /1.68 l water
1 medium chopped red onion
1 lb. /454 g dried black beans, rinsed, cleaned, and soaked overnight
2 tsp /10 ml chili powder
1 chopped red bell pepper
¼ cup /240ml fresh cilantro
1 28-oz. /784 g can diced tomatoes

1 tsp /5 ml coriander powder
Toppings:
Avocado
Lime wedges
Thinly sliced green onions
Cilantro

Instructions:
Add all ingredients except salt to the slow cooker.
Stir.
Set for nine hours on low.
After the beans are soft, add salt.
Remove chipotles and cinnamon stick.
Spoon into bowls and serve with toppings of your choice.

Scrumptious Hot Chocolate with Coconut Milk

Ingredients:
½ cups of unsweetened almond milk
10 tablespoons of coconut milk powder

1 ½ cup of filtered water

6 drops of stevia

5 tablespoon of raw cacao powder

cinnamon

marshmallows

1 ½ tablespoon of agave

Procedure:

Using a medium sized sauce pan, mix all of your ingredients together.

Make sure you keep the heat on low and whisk until you remove all the lumps.

Adjust the sweetness if preferred and serve it topped with marshmallows.

Mouth Watering Alkaline Diet Mexican Scrambled Eggs

INGREDIENTS:

2 organic eggs

Sprinkling of black Pepper

Pinch of Himalayan pink salt

Small handful of roughly chopped coriander

½ avocado

Juice of 1/2 a lemon

Finely chopped fresh chilies to taste

INSTRUCTIONS:

•Whisk the egg with salt and pepper in a bowl.

•Heat a saucepan on medium flame and pour the eggs.

•Stir gently until the eggs are slightly underdone and then remove from the flame.

•Mix coriander in the scrambled egg and sprinkle the chillies.

•Sprinkle lemon juice on the sliced avocado.

•Serve the scrambled eggs and avocado with toast.

Heavenly Red Pepper and Corn Chowder

Servings: **4 - 6**
Prep Time: 30 minutes

Ingredients:
Pepper
Salt
2 tbsp. /30 ml olive oil
4 cups /.95 L frozen sweet corn kernels, divided
½ tsp /2 ½ ml paprika
1 medium chopped red bell pepper
1 tsp /5 ml cumin
3 medium chopped Yukon Gold potatoes
1 medium chopped onion
1 cup /240 ml almond or coconut milk
1/8 tsp /7/8 ml cayenne pepper
4 cups /.95 L vegetable broth
Topping:
Corn kernels
Chopped scallions
Chopped red bell pepper
Instructions:
Heat oil in a pan.
Add onion and cook until soft.
Place in slow cooker with bell pepper, a cup of corn, potatoes, spices, and broth.

Cook for nine hours on low.

After the potatoes are soft, puree everything with an immersion blender.

Stir in 3 cups of corn and almond or soy milk.

Cook an additional 30 minutes on low until warm.

Add pepper and salt to taste.

Serve with toppings of your choice.

Irresistible Spring Pea and Edame Bread Spread

Ingredients:

1 ½ cup of fresh peas

1 ½ cup of edame beans

½ teaspoon of salt

1/3 cup of extra virgin olive oil + some extra

3 stems of fresh mint

Juice from one lime

Lime Zest

Procedure:

Place your edame beans in boiling water for about 4 minutes until it becomes bright green.

Removes them and run the beans under cold water.

Repeat the same for your peas except only leave them in for a minute.

Once done, place both in a food processor and combine until it gets evenly mixed. Don't puree completely.

Add some seasoning and serve in a bowl. A drizzle of olive oil and mint leaf garnish should top it off nicely.

Now that you've got easy to prepare recipes for your everyday breakfast, let's talk lunch. Fast foods are definitely part of your options so, what to do? Prepare it beforehand and take it with you!

Delicious Alkaline Diet Warm Vegan Protein Smoothie

INGREDIENTS:

1 cup boiling water

1 tsp. raw cacao

1 banana

1 scoop of vegan protein powder

¼ cup of gluten free oats

INSTRUCTIONS:

•Place all the ingredients in a blender and blend.

•Check the consistency. If too thick add ½ cup of water.

•Pour in a glass and serve.

Tasty Farro Chili

 Servings: **6 - 8**

Ingredients:

Pepper

3 cups /720 ml low-sodium vegetable broth

Himalayan Salt

1 ½ tbsp. /22.5 ml chili powder

1 15 oz. /420 g can pinto beans, rinsed and drained

2-14oz cans //784 g fire-roasted tomatoes, diced

1 chopped green pepper

1 pkg. sliced mushrooms

1 15 oz. /420 g can black beans, rinsed and drained

1 chopped orange pepper

2 tsp /10 ml garlic powder

1 medium chopped red onion

1 15 oz. /420 g can kidney beans, rinsed and drained

2 tsp /10 ml cumin

1 cup /240 ml farro, rinsed and drained

1 to 3 chipotle peppers in adobo sauce, chopped

Toppings:

Sliced green onions

Cilantro

Avocado

Instructions:

Add all ingredients to the slow cooker. Stir.

Set for eight hours on low.

Veggies should be tender and liquid slightly thickened.

Season with pepper and salt.

Serve with toppings of your choice.

Yummy Raw Zucchini Noodles with Pesto

Ingredients:

6 pieces of 8 inch zucchinis, peeled

1 cup of basil leaves

Celtic sea salt

3 tablespoons of raw hemp hearts

¼ cup of pine nuts or raw cashews

1 clove of garlic, crushed

¼ cup of olive oil

Procedure:

Using your spiral slicer, trim the ends of your zucchini in order to make it line up evenly. Slowly wind it and carefully collect the spaghetti like noodles that would be pushing through the openings on the blade.

For fettuccine like noodles, (and if you have no spiral slicer) you can use a simple peeler. Just be careful and mind the thickness.

Pesto Sauce:

Combine your olive oil, basil, garlic, nuts and sea salt in a blender. Combine this until you achieve the right consistency. Add more oil if needed.

Toss this with your noodles and serve as is to keep noodles nice and crunchy.

Scrumptious Alkaline Diet Fall Apple Fritters

INGREDIENTS:

6 oz. thinly sliced apple

½ tsp. ground cinnamon

¼ tsp. ground ginger

3 tbsp. water

1 oz. rice flour

1 tbsp. coconut oil

2 organic eggs

2 tbsp. agave syrup

INSTRUCTIONS:

•Place the apple, cinnamon, water and ground ginger on a pan on a medium flame for 4 minutes.

- Remove from the heat and keep to cool.
- On cooling, add the rice flour and beaten eggs to the apples.
- Heat a non-stick pan and apply coconut oil onto the pan.
- Ladle some quantity of the mixture into the pan and spread evenly and thickly.
- Cook until the pan side of the pancake is golden brown and you can move the fritter with a spatula.
- Flip it over with the spatula and leave it until done.
- Make fritters with the remaining batter, in the same manner.
- Drizzle with a small amount of syrup, sprinkle cinnamon and serve.

Mouth Watering Vegetable Barley Soup

Servings: **6**
Ingredients:
Pepper

Salt

1 small bunch Swiss chard

8 sprigs fresh thyme

½ cup /120 ml barley (not the quick-cooking kind)

2 medium parsnips, chopped

1 small chopped rutabaga

2 celery stalks, chopped

1 large chopped onion

1 clove garlic, minced

Instructions:

Tie thyme with butcher's twine.

Add 8 cups water, barley, thyme, rutabaga, onion, garlic, celery, parsnips, pepper, and salt.

Cover. Set for 6 hours on low.

Make sure that the barley is tender.

When there is 10 minutes left on the timer, take out the thyme. Turn to high. Add Swiss chard, cover and cook until tender about 5 minutes.

Heavenly Mini Roasted Veggie Skewers with Garlic Basil Dip

Ingredients:

1 sweet white onion

2 red peppers

3 zucchinis

3 cloves of crushed garlic

12 cherry tomatoes

¼ cup of olive oil

Sea salt

12 pieces of skewers

For the dip:

2 cloves of garlic

1 cup of zucchini

½ a cup of extra virgin olive oil

½ cup of raw pistachio nuts

16 basil leaves

½ teaspoon of sea salt

Procedure:

Preheat your oven to 400F.

Combine our oil and garlic, set this aside.

Skewer your veggies, make sure there's a uniform pattern. Set aside.

Baste this well with the garlic oil, spreading the garlic bits onto your vegetable pieces.

Sprinkle some sea salt over it.

Roast for about 15 minutes.

For your dip, simply mix all of your dip ingredients in a blender/food processor until it becomes creamy. Add more olive oil if needed.

Irresistible Alkaline Diet Superfood Acai Blend

INGREDIENTS:

10 ½ oz. frozen strawberries, slightly thawed

2 frozen sliced bananas

4 tbsp. acai powder

1 cup of unsweetened almond milk

2 tbsp. of soaked nuts or seeds

Topping:

fresh fruit, sliced

hemp seeds

bee pollen

Goji berries

2 tsp. of clear honey (preferably unheated), optional

INSTRUCTIONS:

•Place the milk, frozen fruits and the acai powder in a high speed blender.

•Add the soaked nuts and blend till creamy.

•Transfer the creamy acai mixture into bowls and serve topped with sliced fruits, hemp seeds, bee pollen, Goji berries and a little honey.

Delicious Vegetable Stew

Servings: **6**

Ingredients:

Pepper

Salt

1 zucchini, chopped

4 large carrots, sliced diagonally in 2-inch pieces

¼ tsp /1 ¼ ml red pepper flakes

1 15 oz. can /420 g chickpeas, drained

2 medium turnips, peeled and chopped into 1-inch cubes

½ tsp /2 ½ ml cumin

1 large diced onion

1 cup /240 ml vegetable broth

2 cloves minced garlic

1 14 oz. can /392 g diced tomatoes

Instructions:

Add tomatoes and liquid, garlic, onion, turnips, carrots, broth, pepper flakes, cumin, and salt to the slow cooker.

Set for six hours on low.

At the end of six hours, stir in the chickpeas and zucchini.

Cook for another hour. Taste and adjust seasonings if needed.

Tasty Sprouted Grain Wrap with Chipotle Dip

Ingredients:

1 peeled parsnip

2 medium sized beets

1 yellow beet

1 large sweet potato

4 tablespoons of olive oil

1 teaspoon salt

Mixed greens

6 sprouted grain tortilla wraps
Fresh pea shoots
Chipotle Dip
Procedure:
Toss all of your veggies with oil and salt but keep your red beets separate.

Once done, spoon these into your baking sheet, sprinkling the red beets on top. Make sure it's parchment lined.

Roast this in a preheated oven (350 degrees) for about 25 minutes until it becomes slightly tender. Remove and allow to cool.

Over your wrap pile your greens and spoon some of the roasted roots down its center. Add some of your chipotle dip on top before sprinkling some of the pea shoots.

Serve with extra dip and some avocado.

Yummy Alkaline Diet Coconut Berry Porridge

INGREDIENTS:

1 cup gluten free rolled oats

1.5 cups water

2 tbsp. coconut oil

1 tbsp. coconut yoghurt (optional)

1/2 a cup of almond milk

For the Blueberry Sauce:

1/2 a cup of blueberries

2 tbsp. water

Toppings:

Handful of fresh raspberries

1/4 cup of warm toasted almonds, roughly chopped

Sprinkling of bee pollen (optional)

INSTRUCTIONS:

• Pre-heat the oven to 175 degrees Celsius and toast the almonds for 5 minutes.

•In a medium sized pan, add the oats and water and cook on a low flame until all the water is absorbed.

•Add the coconut oil and stir until mixed well.

•Then add coconut milk and yogurt and set aside.

•For the blueberry sauce place the berries and water in a pan and simmer on a medium flame until the berries break down and you get a thick sauce.
•Stir the blueberry sauce through the porridge.
•Transfer the porridge into bowls and serve topped with the berries and nuts.

Scrumptious Vegan Jambalaya

Servings: **4**
Prep Time: 10 minutes
Ingredients:
Pepper
Himalayan Salt
6 oz. /168 g soy chorizo
¼ tsp /1 ¼ ml cayenne pepper
2 cups /480 ml cooked rice
½ tsp /2 ½ ml paprika
1 ½ cups /360 ml vegetable broth
1 chopped bell pepper
½ medium chopped onion

2 10 oz. cans /560 ml diced tomatoes with green chilies

1 cup /240 ml sliced okra

1 chopped celery stalk

2 cloves minced garlic

Instructions:

Add the chorizo to a skillet. Cook until browned and add to the crockpot.

Add the garlic, celery, onion, okra, and bell pepper to the crockpot. Pour the tomatoes with their juices and broth over the top.

Add spices and stir. Set for six hours on low.

Add cooked rice. Give it a good stir. Serve and enjoy.

Mouth Watering Rainbow Salad with Avocado and Meyer Lemon Dressing

Ingredients:

Baby spinach and arugula greens

1 yellow beet

2 carrots

6 slices of yellow pepper

¼ red onion

Pea shots

Micro greens or sprouts

1 avocado

Chopped pistachios

Dressing:

1 avocado

2 Meyer lemons

1 ½ teaspoon of red onion

6 fresh dill

6 basil leaves

1/8 teaspoon of sea salt

1/3 cup cold pressed extra virgin olive oil

3 drops of stevia

Procedure:

Prepare your serving bowls.

In each of them place a generous amount of your arugula.

Top this with beets and surround that with other veggies. Make sure that everything is layered properly.

Add your micro greens, pea shoots and top this with your pistachios.

For the dressing, simply process all of the ingredients in a blender. Make sure it reaches a creamy consistency before pouring it in a separate container.

Heavenly Alkaline Diet Raw Buckwheat Porridge

INGREDIENTS:

3 oz. raw buckwheat kernels

1 ½ gluten free porridge oats

2 tsp. golden linseeds

4 dates

Water to cover

1 banana

2 ½ blueberries

2tsp acai berry powder

3tbsp water

INSTRUCTIONS:

•Mix the buckwheat kernels, oats, linseeds and dates.

•Cover in water and soak for an hour.

•Once the buckwheat has softened, drain the water.

•Transfer to a high speed blender along with the banana and pulse until you get a porridge like texture.

•Place the blueberries, water and the acai berry powder onto a pan and simmer till the berries breakdown to form a thick sauce.

•Place the porridge into bowls and top it with the blueberry sauce.

Irresistible Indian Stew

Servings: **2**
Ingredients:
Pepper
Salt
2 ½ cups /600 ml cooked lentils
Juice of one lemon
1 tsp /5 ml garam masala
1 sweet potato, peeled and diced
2/3 cup /160 ml vegetable broth
½ tsp /2 ½ ml ground ginger

1 yellow bell pepper, chopped

¼ tsp /1 ¼ ml cayenne pepper

1 medium chopped onion

1 tbsp. /30 ml coriander

3 – 4 cloves minced garlic

1 15 oz. /420 g tomato sauce

1 tsp /5 ml turmeric

2 tsp /10 ml paprika

2 tsp /10 ml cumin

Instructions:

Add all ingredients to the slow cooker.

Set for three hours on high.

When sweet potatoes are tender, serve with brown rice.

Delicious Raw Cranberry Pie to Go

Ingredients:

1 organic pear

2 cups of raw organic cranberries

¼ wedge of orange (keep the skin)

Juice from half an orange

½ cup of raw almonds

6 dates

½ cup of raw pecans
¼ teaspoon of cinnamon
1/8 teaspoon allspice
1/8 teaspoon ground cloves
2 tablespoon of maple syrup
½ a teaspoon of vanilla
1 cup of untoasted buckwheat
Procedure:
For the base:
Soak your buckwheat using filtered water for half an hour. Rinse and drain properly.

Combine this with ¼ teaspoon of cinnamon and the orange juice. Add your maple syrup and half a teaspoon of vanilla. Set this aside.

For the filling:
Using your food processor, mix your cranberries, your orange, dates, a teaspoon of cinnamon, cloves, all spice and half and teaspoon of vanilla.

Make sure this is blended well then set aside.

For the pie topping:

Place 2 dates, pecans, almonds and ¼ teaspoon of cinnamon in a food processor.
Blend until it becomes crumbly.
Now fill your jar layer by layer. Buckwheat bottom, then 2 scoops of the cranberry mixture and topped with the nut crumbles.
Top this with some fresh cranberry and seal the lid.

Tasty Alkaline Diet Breakfast Turmeric Omelette

INGREDIENTS:
3 organic eggs
2cm of fresh turmeric, finely grated
Pinch of Himalayan salt
1 tbsp. sunflower oil
1 spring onion, finely sliced
¼ courgette, grated
1 tbsp. chopped parsley
INSTRUCTIONS:
•Whisk the eggs in a bowl along with the grated turmeric and salt.

•Heat a non stick frying pan and spread sunflower oil.

•Pour the egg mixture onto the pan and sprinkle the courgette, spring onion and parsley.

•Cook for 3-4 minutes until the edges are done and the center is not too runny.

•With the spatula gently flip the egg and cook on the other side.

•Serve with salad and toast.

Yummy White Bean Soup

Servings: **10**

Ingredients:

Pepper

1 lb. /454 g dry white beans of choice, rinsed and sorted

1 – 2 tsp /5 – 10 ml dried dill

2 quarts /1.9 L vegetable broth

Salt

1 medium chopped onion

1 pound /454 g frozen, sliced carrots

1 cup /240 ml chopped sun-dried tomatoes*

4 cloves garlic, smashed and peeled

3 – 4 tbsp. /45 – 60 ml fresh parsley, minced

2 medium potatoes, diced

Instructions:

Add the potatoes, beans, garlic, onion, broth, pepper, and salt to the slow cooker. Set for eight hours on low.

When beans are soft but not totally mushy, add dill, tomatoes, and carrots. Taste to see if you need any additional salt or pepper. Cook an additional 30 minutes.

*Look for dehydrated sun-dried tomatoes instead of the canned ones in oil. They are cheaper. Just rehydrate them in some water prior to putting them in the crockpot. You could add the liquid from the tomatoes to the soup for added flavor.

Scrumptious Dairy Free Cherry, Avocado and Coconut Ice Cream

Ingredients:

2 cups of cherries + 6 more, finely chopped

½ of a large avocado

1 400ml organic full fat coconut milk

1/3 cup of cashews

10 soft dried dates

Juice of half a lemon

2/3 cup of filtered water

1/3 cup of cashews, soaked and drained

2 tablespoon agave syrup

2 tablespoon beet juice (for color)

Finely chopped dark chocolate

Procedure:

Using a high speed blender, combine 2 cups of cherries, avocado, coconut milk, water, cashews, dates and lemon juice.

Blend this until it becomes creamy. Taste it for sweetness before adding your agave.

Stir your chocolate and chopped cherries into this mixture.

Transfer this to your ice cream maker and follow the instructions.

You can also choose to freeze this overnight.

Garnish with a few more chopped cherries before serving.

Mouth Watering Alkaline Diet Poached Plums

INGREDIENTS:

10 ½ oz. plums

1/4 tsp. agave powder

4 whole star anise

1/4 cup water

2 heaped tbsp. coyo coconut yoghurt

INSTRUCTIONS:

•Cut the plums into half and remove the pips.

•Put all ingredients onto a saucepan and leave to simmer on medium heat, until the plums are soft and begin splitting.

•Serve with delicious syrup or with coyo coconut yogurt.

Conclusion

Congrats! You made it to the end of the book. I hope you have found this book useful and full of all the valuable information you will need to get started cooking.

The next step is to start making these alkaline diet recipes and be on your way to living a healthier lifestyle!

Finally, if you have found tremendous benefit from this book, leaving a review would be fantastic!

Part – 2

48

Introduction

This book contains proven steps and strategies on how to lose weight using one of the most basic yet unique methods on the market today... eating for your body rather than against it.

Not many people realize how much damage they are doing to their bodies by eating foods that are highly processed, or foods that are simply poor choices. When it comes to weight loss and your body, you need to focus on nutrition, variety, and food that your body can actually use.

So many people focus on the wrong things in their diets, including:

Convenience – prepackaged foods you can find in the frozen or refrigerated section of the grocery stores. Foods you only need to add one or two ingredients to before you have a meal.

Calories – restricting foods which only allow you to eat a small portion of whatever it is you like, no matter how hungry you are or how you feel.

Carbohydrates – diets which avoid carbohydrates... including fruits and vegetables... in favor of protein and fats.

Fats – the low-fat way of eating still manages to hang onto our society, though it really is another way to eat foods that aren't in their natural state.

Name brands – foods that are endorsed by a certain chef, nutritionist, or TV network.

Diet endorsed – foods that bear the name of a specific diet (Atkins diet, Beach Body diet, etc.)

Or other things along these lines – virtually any diet that promises you the results you want without any real basis behind it. Diets that focus on foods that are basically ready to go straight out of the package. Diets that are way too easy to be considered healthy.

People get so hung up on who is endorsing their diet rather than what the diet can actually do for them, or perhaps more importantly, what the diet is doing to their bodies.

When you are trying to lose weight, you need to give your body the proper nutrition it requires while controlling your portion sizes and eating real foods. I don't believe in throwing back a bunch of supplements and vitamins, I believe in using your food to get the nutrition you need.

And with the Alkaline diet, you are doing that very thing. This diet focuses on the acidity and PH levels of your body, with the end goal of keeping your PH in balance as much as possible.

You see, your body knows how to process foods, and it knows how to maintain a proper weight... under the right circumstances.

The Alkaline diet allows real foods which do not interact with your bodies acidity, keeping the acid-base relationship within your body as close to perfect as possible.

Why would you want to maintain this relationship?

When the acidity of your body gets out of balance, it's easy for disease to creep in. Keeping your body in balance has been shown to be excellent for your heart health, your kidney health, as well as your liver health.

There is some supporting evidence which shows that this diet is could be a great option for preventing cancer, and could possibly even help those who have been diagnosed with cancer.

Not to mention... the weight benefits.

When you quit eating processed foods, foods that are high in sugars, foods which are high in sodium, and similar foods, your body is able to get rid of the ill affects these things have.

When this happens, your body is better able to process the foods you put into it, allowing you to utilize the food as energy rather than fat... causing you to shed the pounds. What makes this even better is the fact that you can lose weight without stress or spending hours in the gym, it's a natural side effect of changing your eating patterns.

So which foods are allowed, and which ones am I supposed to avoid?

With the alkaline diet, you will be eating as many real and whole foods as you want, with the exception of meats, some grains, and dairy.

There are minor exceptions in all diets, but as a general rule of thumb, it's the canned foods, meats, dairy (milk, cheese, etc.) sugary foods, caffeine, alcohol, eggs, and several grains ought to be avoided as these will raise your body's acidity.

This diet takes some time to get used to, but with books like these, you will be on the right track in no time. The recipes are simple and easy to follow, they aren't going to take you all day to put together, and they are delicious. Fall in love with each and every one, and mix and match to enjoy them all month long.

You deserve to weigh what you want to weigh and love the body you're in, and this is the perfect place to start.

are for clarifying purposes only and are the owned by the owners themselves, not affiliated with this document.

Chapter 1 – Easy Alkaline Breakfasts for the Busy Person

Breakfast is the most important meal of the day, and when you are concerned about where your food comes from, it can be a challenge to find foods that meet your standards.

In a world that thrives on convenience, you know that breakfast is one of the most processed meals of the day. Whether people are eating cereal and poptarts to pre-packaged sandwiches, but you want something that is natural and whole.

With these recipes, you have found the answer. Indulge in breakfasts that will maintain your body's PH levels and help you lose weight while keeping you full until lunch time.

Medieval Smoothies

What you will need:

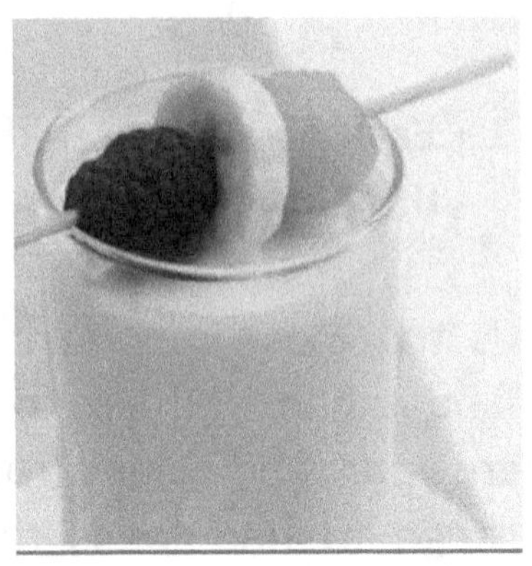

2 dragon fruit

2 cups coconut milk

1 small can coconut cream

1 tablespoon agave syrup

1 teaspoon vanilla

Ice

Directions:

Remove the skin from the dragon fruit and add to your blender. Open the can of coconut cream and add to the blender next, then add the rest of the ingredients (except for the ice).

Turn on your blender and blend well, then add the ice a few cubes at a time, until you reach your desired consistency.

Chicken Little Pancakes

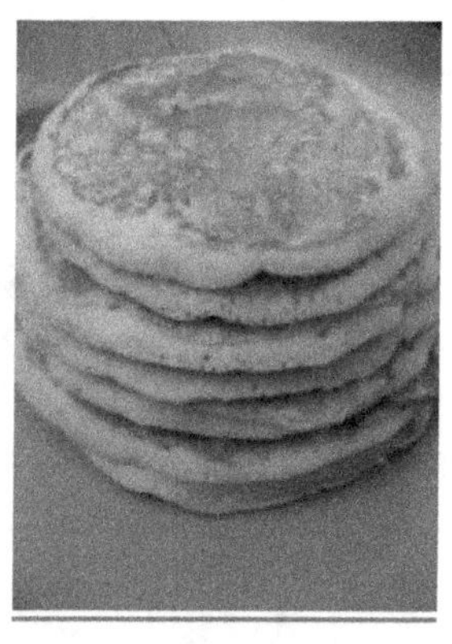

What you will need:

1 cup chickpea flour

1 cup coconut milk

Himalayan salt

2 tablespoons baking soda

Splash of vanilla

2 tablespoons agave nectar

Directions:

Combine the dry ingredients one bowl, and the wet ingredients in another, then combine all ingredients with a whisk in the same bowl.

Preheat a griddle on the stove, then use a ladle to divide the pancakes into 4 to 6 portions.

Cook for roughly 3 minutes on each side, until they are golden brown. Serve immediately.

Wonderful World of Green Smoothies

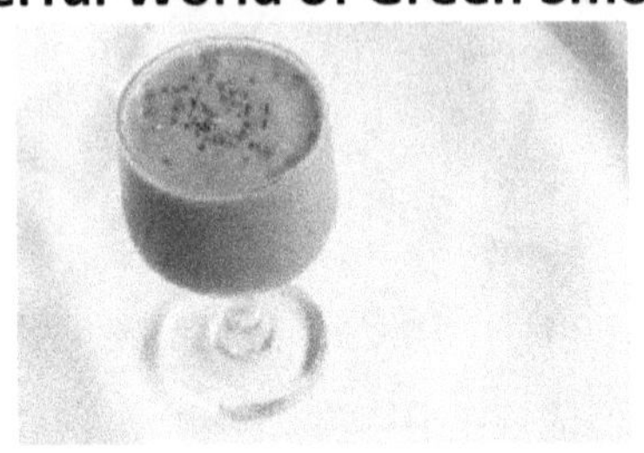

What you will need:

1 cup spinach

1 cup kale

2 cups almond milk

1 tablespoon peanut butter

Splash of alcohol free vanilla

1 teaspoon flax seeds

1 teaspoon hemp seeds

Ice cubes

Directions:

Tear the spinach and kale into smaller pieces and place them in your blender. Add the almond milk, and blend. Add the peanut butter next, then blend well once more.

Finish with the vanilla and flax seed, and turn on to high. Once the smoothie is completely blended, begin adding in the ice cubes, a few cubes at a time, until you get the consistency you are looking for. Serve immediately.

Powerful Protein Toast

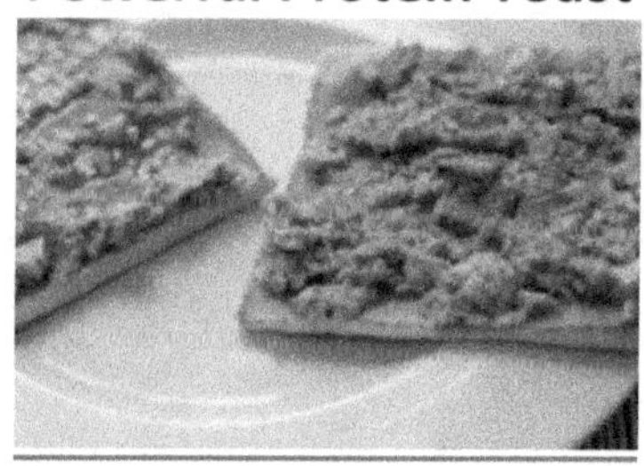

What you will need:

2 slices sprouted whole wheat bread

½ cup edamame

½ cup peas

1 teaspoon garlic powder

1/3 cup olives

Himalayan salt

Coconut oil

Directions:

If you are using frozen peas or edamame, cook them and drain them. Use a fork to smash in a bowl and combine until they are a smooth paste. Set aside.

Heat a pan over medium heat on the stove, and melt the coconut oil in the pan. You don't need much, just enough to toast your whole wheat bread.

As the pan is heating, chop your olives, then combine the a olives with the pea mix and garlic powder.

By now your toast should be done, remove from the pan on the stove and spread the peas on top.

Enjoy immediately.

Chapter 2 – Excellent Alkaline Lunches for Those on the Go

Lunch can be a difficult meal to fit into your day, regardless of the lifestyle you live. Whether you are trying to balance a busy work schedule, kids, life in general, or all the above, you know that lunch time is a meal that's more often forgotten about than it is enjoyed.

But when you are on the alkaline diet, you can take the time to enjoy your lunch, knowing that you are doing the right thing for your body and your health. No one likes to feel hungry, and with this diet and your balanced body, you will watch the weight fall off as you keep full.

Enjoy each of these lunches throughout the week, then mix and match to keep the flow going all month long.

Collie Ranch Wings

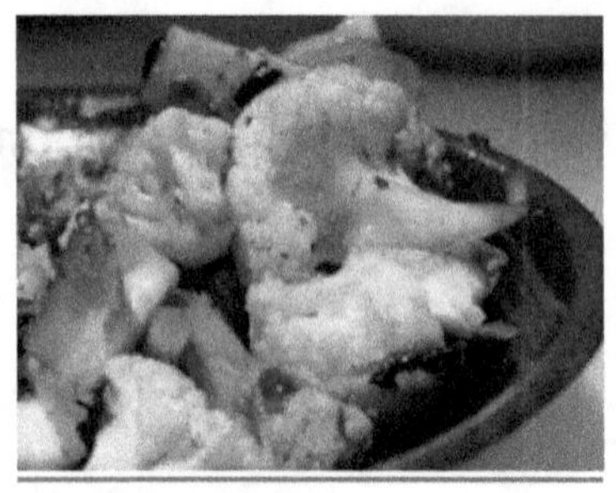

What you will need:

1 head cauliflower

Pepper

Salt

½ cup almond milk

¾ cup almond flour

1 tablespoon cayenne pepper

Directions:

Preheat oven to 300 degrees F.

Cut your head of cauliflower into larger pieces, about the size of chicken wings.

In a separate dish, combine salt, pepper, cayenne, and the almond flour, and pour the almond milk into another dish.

Dip the cauliflower first in the almond milk, then in the almond flour, and lay on a baking sheet.

Bake in the oven for 10 minutes, turn, then bake another 1o minutes, and let stand for a few minutes before enjoying.

Avocado Toast Done Right

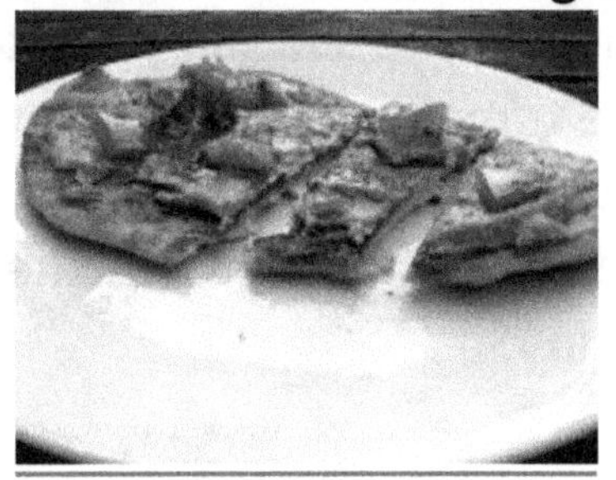

What you will need:

2 slices sprouted whole wheat bread

1 avocado

1 tomato

Himalayan sea salt

Garlic powder

1 tablespoon olive oil

1 tablespoon coconut oil

Directions:

Heat the coconut oil in a pan on the stove over medium heat, and toast the bread in this oil.

You will use only the coconut oil for the bread, so be sure you spread the coconut oil to last for all 4 sides of bread.

As the bread is toasting, slice your avocado, then smash it in a dish with the olive oil and sea salt to taste.

Cut the tomato, then remove the bread from the pan and spread the avocado spread across it. Top with the tomato, and enjoy!

Crunchy Kale Tacos

2 cups chopped kale
1 cup chopped almonds
1/3 cup pine nuts
1 teaspoon turmeric
1 tablespoon garlic
Himalayan sea salt
Splash of water
Sprouted tortillas

Directions:
Chop the kale into smaller pieces, then combine with the almonds and pine nuts.
In a separate dish, combine the spices with a splash of water, adding a little extra

water to make it more of a dressing than a paste. Add the kale and toss together. Divide the kale between two tortillas, and enjoy.

World's Easiest Broccoli Soup

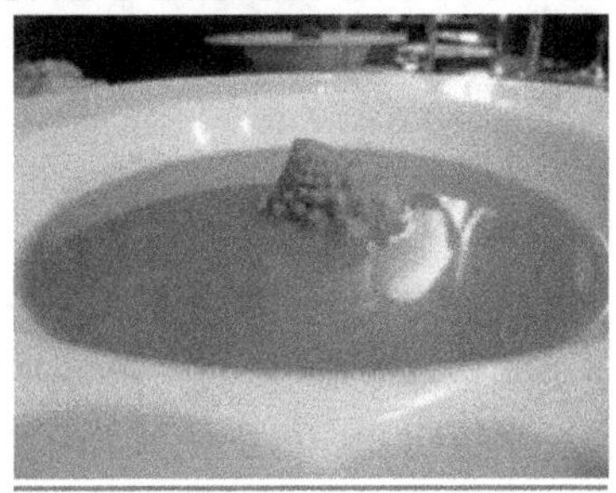

What you will need:

1 onion

1 cup broccoli

1 cup cauliflower

1 carrot

1 can coconut cream

½ cup coconut milk

Salt

Pepper

Garlic powder

Water

Directions:

Chop all the veggies as small as you can get them, then place in a pot with all the other ingredients and 2 cups water.

Bring to a boil and keep an eye on the water, you may need to add more as the veggies cook. Once they are soft, reduce the heat.

Take your emulsifier and blend the soup well, continuing to mix until it is completely smooth.

Season to taste, and let simmer for a few more minutes. Enjoy!

Chapter 3 – Excellent Anytime Alkaline Dinners

Who doesn't like to sit down to a wonderful dinner after a long day on your feet? Who has the time to slave over a stove and prepare an elaborate meal with the schedule you keep?

But who wants to sacrifice taste and nutrition for convenience?

Dinner can be a struggle for many busy people, because it's hard to find the time to put together a dish that is healthy and tastes good but doesn't take hours to make. When you have a busy schedule, it's hard enough to find time to eat dinner, let alone make it.

But with the alkaline diet, you will not only get the nutrition and taste you are looking for, but you can enjoy delicious dinners that take less than half an hour to make. Dive into these delicacies any time, and feel good about the food you put into your body.

Winter Wonder Pumpkin Soup

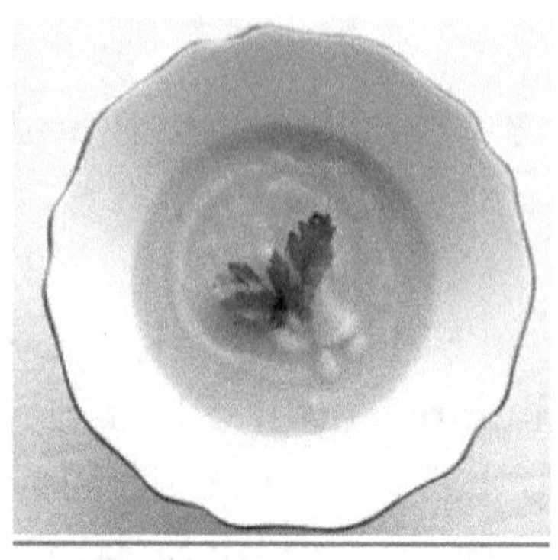

What you will need:

1 onion

4 stalks celery

1 can pumpkin

4 cups veggie broth

4 cups cauliflower florets

1 tablespoon vegetable oil

2 cups coconut milk

Garlic powder

Salt

Pepper

Lemon juice

Parsley flakes

Directions:

Chop the onion into much smaller pieces, then cook in your pot with the oil until they become translucent. You will be making all the soup in this pot, so make sure it's large enough to bring in more ingredients. Slice the celery into thin slices, then chop the cauliflower into as small of pieces as you can get them as well.

Add the celery to the pot next, then the cauliflower. Cook another couple minutes before adding in the pumpkin, coconut milk, and seasonings.

Let all ingredients simmer on the stove for 20 minutes, then use a stick blender and blend until smooth.

If you want the soup thinner, add more coconut milk, otherwise, let simmer until you are ready to enjoy!

World's Best Kabobs

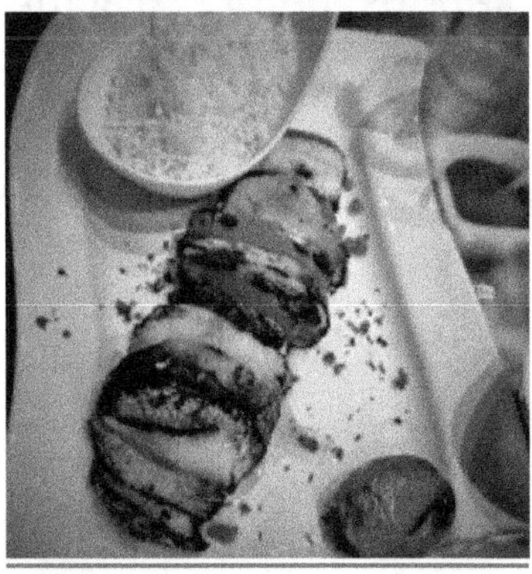

What you will need:

1 red onion

1 red pepper

1 zucchini

2 tablespoons olive oil

Himalayan salt

Pepper

Directions:

Turn your oven on to 400 degrees F, and chop your onion into large pieces. Make sure you leave enough room to use your skewers on your onion, so slice it to form leaflets, and not thin strings.

Slice the red pepper and the zucchini the same, then layer on the skewers.

Combine the salt and olive oil, then drizzle over the kabobs before placing them in your oven. Bake for 10 minutes on one side, then flip the skewers over and bake for another 10 minutes on the other side. Enjoy!

Busy Night Skillet

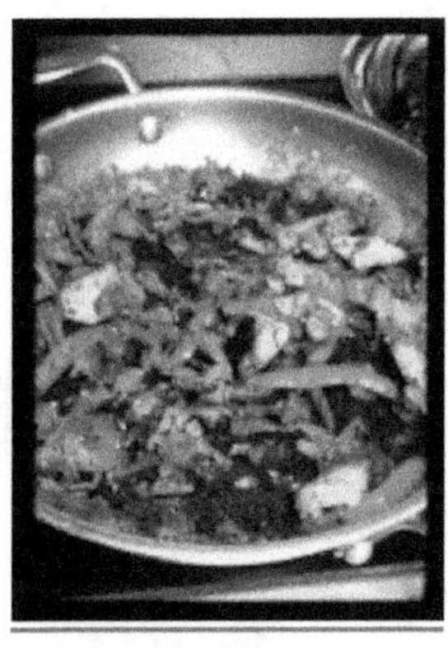

What you will need:

    1 cup cooked brown rice
6 cups vegetable oil
1 tablespoon olive oil
1 red onion
2 green peppers
1 tomato
1 cup fresh green beans
    1 cup chickpeas
½ cup edamame
Salt
Pepper
1 can coconut cream

Directions:
Chop the peppers, the tomato, and the onion and add to a deep skillet on the

stove. Turn the skillet on to medium high and add the olive oil.

Add the rice (already cooked), the green beans, and the edamame.

Open your can of chickpeas and add this next, and stir. Let these cook for 5 minutes before you add the rest of the ingredients.

Season to taste, and add extra water if it appears to dry.

Allow to simmer on the stove for another 10 minutes, until all the veggies are tender.

Serve immediately.

Texas Munch

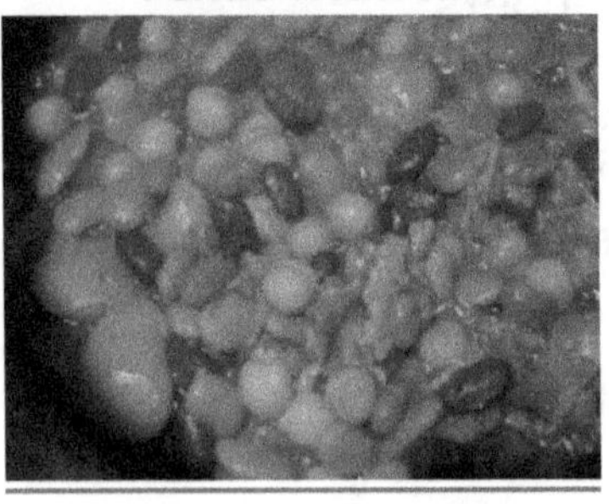

What you will need:

1 cup black beans

1 cup pinto beans

1 cup frozen corn

1 onion

1 can tomato paste

Garlic powder

1 tomato

1 can olives

Himalayan salt

Taco seasoning

1 tablespoon lime juice

Directions:

Thaw the corn and cook the beans if they aren't cooked and ready to go. Chop the onion. Combine all ingredients in a skillet on the stove and turn on to medium heat. Season to taste with salt, pepper, and taco seasoning, then let continue to simmer for 10 to 15 minutes.

Serve immediately.

Chapter 4 – Alkaline Desserts that Actually Help You Lose Weight

Dessert is hands down the best meal of the day, and when you are on the Alkaline diet, you can help yourself to seconds! These desserts are the perfect cap to any day of the week, and with them, you can get your sweet cravings under control and still lose the weight you have been wanting to lose.

You have discovered the diet that allows you the best of both worlds. Enjoy both the richness of your favorite meal of the day but still fit into that dress this Christmas... it's the best gift anyone could imagine.

I know it can be tempting when you walk through the store and see all the different pastries and desserts which line the shelves, but trust me, as soon as you taste any one of these delicious desserts here, you will fall in love with the Alkaline style, and won't ever feel tempted to go back.

Eat dessert and still lose weight... sounds like a match made in heaven to me.

Decadent Chocolate "Ice Cream"

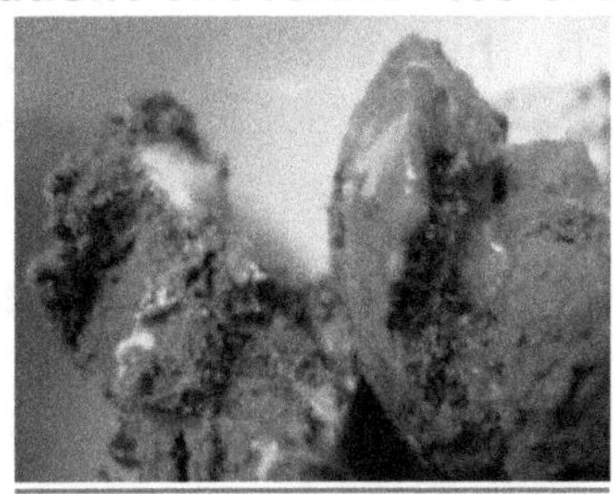

What you will need:

3 tablespoons organic baking cocoa

2 bananas

3 tablespoons raw honey

½ avocado

1 cup blueberries

1 tablespoon chia seeds

1/3 cup almond milk

Vanilla

1 can coconut cream

1 tablespoon chocolate chips

Directions:

Slice the banana and place in a dish in the freezer for at least 2 hours. Once the bananas are frozen, add them to your blender, and combine the milk, honey, and splash of vanilla along with them.

Turn on the blender and blend until they are smooth, then begin adding the other ingredients. Slice the avocado into small pieces and add that next, blending until completely smooth. Once all ingredients are combined, check the consistency.

If you want it creamier and more pudding like, add in more avocado, if you would like it to be more smoothie like, add in the ice cubes.

When you are happy with the consistency, serve and enjoy immediately.

Granny Smith's Favorite Cookies

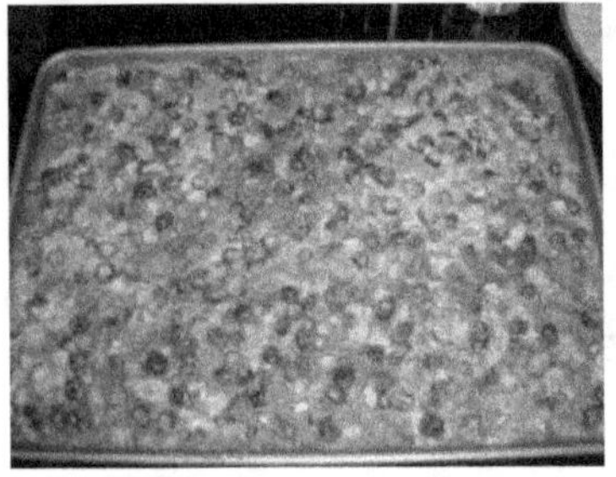

What you will need:

8 figs

1 tablespoon molasses

1 granny smith apple

2 cups almond pulp

Cinnamon

1 teaspoon nutmeg

2 tablespoons agave nectar

1/3 cup dried cranberries

1/3 cup raisins

Directions:

Preheat your oven to 180 degrees F.

In a food processor, combine all ingredients. The dough should be crumbly, but still maintain some moisture. Press this into a shallow baking dish lined with parchment paper.

Place in the oven and bake for 20 -30 minutes.

Let cool for 8-10 minutes, then cut bars into cookie portions.

Store in the refrigerator for up to 1 week.

Perfectly Pleasant Popper Corn

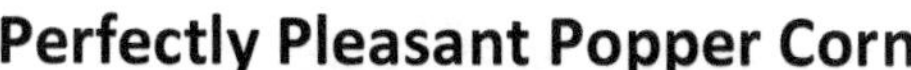

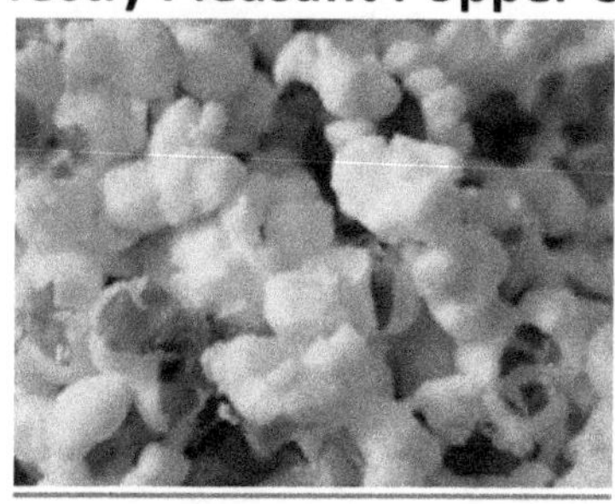

What you will need:

4 tablespoons popcorn kernels

1 tablespoon coconut oil

Himalayan salt

1 tablespoon honey

1 teaspoon organic cacao

Directions:

If you have an old fashioned popper, heat the oil on the stove for a few minutes before adding the kernels. Stir the kernels, letting them pop as they do, and once they have finished popping, remove from heat.

If you do not have an old fashioned popper, heat the oil in a pot (with a lid) on the stove, and add the kernels to the pot. Use hot pads and gently shake the pot as the kernels are popping, and once the last one is popped, remove from heat and place on a cookie sheet.

Drizzle the honey over the popcorn, then dust with the cacao.

Serve immediately.

Seductively Sweet Chocolate Chia Pudding

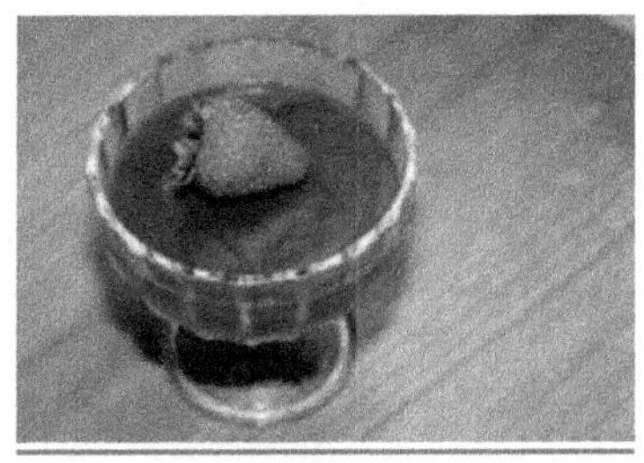

What you will need:

1 cup almond milk

3 tablespoons honey

2 tablespoons chia seeds

2 tablespoons dried, pitted cherries

1 teaspoon organic coco powder (reserve)

3 tablespoons organic cocoa powder

Directions:

In a dish, start by combining the honey and 3 tablespoons of cocoa powder. Hold back the rest of the cocoa powder in reserve for the rest of the recipe.

Once combined, stir in the chia seeds, then the pitted cherries. Your mix ought to be rather thick by now.

Add in the almond milk, and use a whisk to stir thoroughly. It may be a challenge to get all the lumps out, but you will get it

with some persistence and vigorous stirring.
Once you have this thoroughly combined, place in your fridge overnight, or if you are making this in the morning, place in the fridge for the rest of the day.
After 12 hours, your pudding should be thick enough to enjoy. Give it a stir, and you are ready to indulge!

Chapter 5 – Alkaline Snacks

It doesn't seem to matter what time of day you manage to squeeze in breakfast, or when you eat lunch. Sometime in the middle of the afternoon or in the middle of the morning, you simply must have that sweet snack.

But, when you are on a diet, you know you have to be careful. You don't want to spend so much time being careful of what you eat to have it all go out the window with the mid-morning hunger.

Thankfully you have plenty of options with the Alkaline diet. From countless fruits and veggies to choose from to quick and easy snack mixes, I have you covered from the middle of the morning the middle of the afternoon.

Breakfast, lunch, and dinner are connected with lovely little snacks in between, so cut loose and have a snack, you will feel better, have better focus, and still see the weight come off within days.

Who knew your transformation could be so easy?

The Bumble Bee Bundle

What you will need:

- 1 apple
- 2 tablespoons peanut butter
- 1 tablespoon raisins
- 1 tablespoon dried blueberries
- 1 tablespoon honey
- 1 teaspoon cocoa powder

Directions:

In a dish, stir together the cocoa powder, honey, blueberries, and raisins with the peanut butter. This mix is going to be thick, but you can get it.

Take a knife next and carefully hollow out the center of an apple, removing the core and seeds.

Spoon the mix you have made into the center of this apple, and enjoy immediately.

Sweets to the Sweet Snowballs

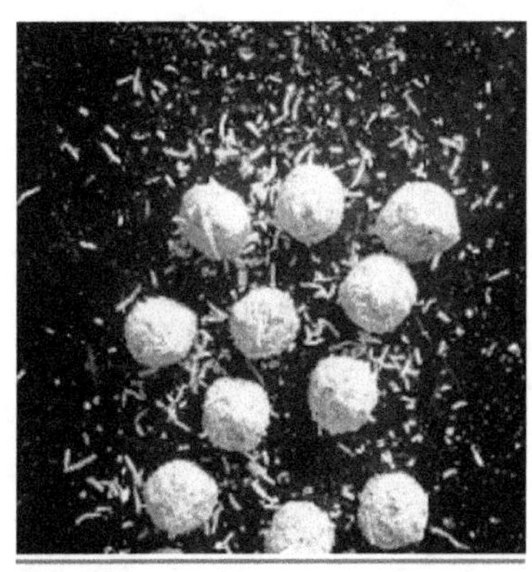

What you will need:

½ cup shredded coconut

1 tablespoon raisins

1 teaspoon crushed almonds

2 tablespoons agave nectar

Directions:

Place the coconut, raisins, and almonds into a bowl. Mix with your hands.

Add the agave nectar, a little at a time, you want the mix to be sticky enough to form into balls, but not so sticky that it falls apart. I recommend you use gloves for this part.

Once you are able, form the coconut mix into 3 balls, and place on a plate in the fridge.

Let set up for 1 to 2 hours, and your sweet snowballs are ready to enjoy.

Matchsticks in Mud

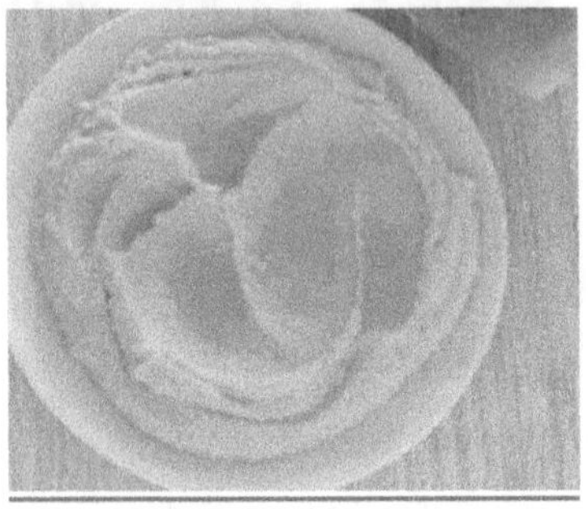

What you will need:

3 celery stalks

½ cup cooked chickpeas

Garlic powder

Pepper

Salt

Lime juice

1 tablespoon coconut milk

Directions:

In a bowl, smash the chickpeas with the coconut milk, and add in a squeeze of lime juice, pepper, garlic powder, and salt to taste.

Use a fork to smash and mix this until you have hummus, then set aside.

Wash the celery, and slice them into lengths, then slice these lengths in half the long way to double the amount you have. Stick the lengths of celery in the hummus to create the matchsticks, and enjoy!

Gone Nutzo

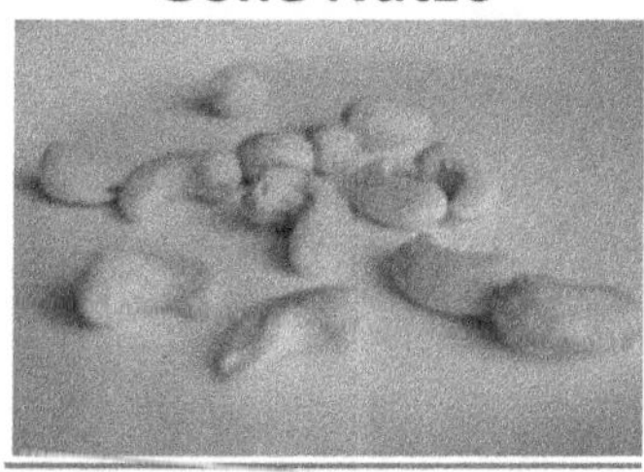

What you will need:

12 almonds

6 cashews

6 brazil nuts

6 hazelnuts

1 tablespoon peanuts

2 teaspoons peanut oil

Cayenne pepper

Himalayan sea salt

Directions:

Preheat your oven to 350 degrees F.

Toss the nuts with the oil in a bowl, then spread on a baking sheet. Season with the

pepper and salt to taste, then place in the oven and bake for 5-10 minutes.
Pull them out of the oven and let stand on a cookie sheet for another 5-10 minutes, and enjoy!

Conclusion

Thank you again for downloading this book!

I hope this book was able to help you to see how many easy things you can make while on the Alkaline diet, and that you can whip them up any day of the week!

The next step is to stick with this diet. There are so many diets out there that promise fast results, and tell you if you go to them for just a few weeks, you will be down to your goal weight, but I warn you, they aren't healthy, and they aren't going to give you the results you want.

With this diet, you can eat all the healthy foods you want, and still lose weight. There's no counting calories, no stressing about how many carbs you had or how many grams of fat you had, and there's no worry about what you had for lunch, because you know you can have as much of dinner as you want, too.

I hope this book was able to show you that snacks and desserts are ok, and that you can still lose the weight you want to lose, even while you enjoy the same kinds of meals you once did.

You may not lose the weight as quickly as other diets promise, but you are losing the weight in a healthy way that will last for the long term, which is much better than dropping pounds simply to lose them.

The recipes in this book are perfect for anything you need, whether you are on a tight schedule and need something fast, you are looking to try something that is new, or you are just curious about this diet and wonder if you can eat foods that taste great while you lose weight.

This book was able to show you all those things, and more, and I hope you keep coming back to try these recipes again and again. There's no end to the combinations you can do, and even adding little adjustments here and there are going to give you entirely different meals that you can enjoy time and time again.

I know with these recipes you are going to reach your best self, and I know you will be happy.

So thank you for downloading this book, and enjoy each recipe you make. You deserve to be happy, and I know if you eat this way, you will be. Now get out there and lose the weight you want to lose, and embrace that life you have been dreaming of.
Good luck!

Thank you and good luck!